# Contents

3

# INTRODUCTION:

In a typical diet, humans have to eat higher amounts of carbohydrates as this acts as energy basis for the body to be able to function appropriately and, less of fat as fats are only stockpiled in the body as a fallback for when the body needs more fuel.

As the body requires more carbohydrates, it processes the food group first, and consequently one feels hungry after a while which is not so in the case of breaking down meals that are very high in fat content.

In the ketogenic diet, this theory is overturned. One will need to eat a higher amount of fats and trick the body into recognizing that it has an insufficient amount of glucose so that it would breakdown the fats first and transform these into energies.

The ketogenic diet first made to know to in the 1920s as a means to control epilepsy in children.

In more recent times, the principles of the ketogenic diet have been enhanced for a highly effective weight loss plan.

The ketogenic diet is high in fat, low in carbohydrates, and is intended to offer adequate protein and calories for a healthy weight.

The vital aim of the diet is to prompt the body to burn fat instead of carbohydrate, which has the effect of fast weight loss.

The high-fat content could cause astonishment and worry in a health-conscious society which associates 'fat' with 'bad.'

Moreover, good fats are healthy and essential as part of a controlled and balanced diet.

High levels of carbohydrates, on the other hand, could cause a spike in blood sugar levels, which can lead to obesity and low energy levels.

CHAPTER ONE:

# What is keto diet

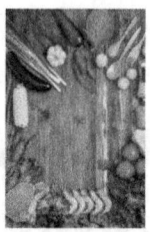

A ketogenic diet for beginners

A keto or ketogenic diet is a very low-carb diet, which could assist you to burn to fat more successfully. Numerous folks have already experienced its many confirmed benefits for weight loss, health, and performance.

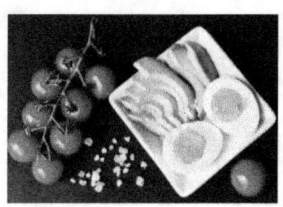

What is the keto diet?

We make it simple to comprehend a keto diet and do it correctly,

What "keto" means

"keto" in a ketogenic diet comes from the fact that it allows the body to make small fuel molecules named "ketones."

This is an another fuel source for the body, used when blood sugar (glucose) is in acute supply.

Ketones are made if you eat very few carbs (that are speedily broken down into blood sugar) and only reasonable amounts of protein (excess protein can also be made to blood sugar).

The liver produces ketones from fat. These ketones then serve as a fuel source all through the body, particularly for the brain.

The brain is a hungry organ that eats lots of energy every day, and it can't run on fat directly. It could only run on glucose... or ketones.

On a ketogenic diet, your whole body switches its fuel supply to run typically on fat, burning fat 24-7. As soon, as insulin levels become very low, fat burning can increase radically.

It becomes easier to get your fat stores to burn them off.

This is splendid, if you're trying to lose weight, however, there are also other less observable benefits, such as less hunger and a stable supply of energy. This might help keep you alert and motivated.

When the body produces ketones, it moves into a metabolic state termed ketosis. The fastest route to get there is by fasting – not eating anything – though nobody can fast forever.

A keto diet, on the other hand, can be eaten for an indefinite period and also results in ketosis. It has several of the benefits of fasting – comprising weight loss – without having to fast.

The ketogenic diet (or keto diet, for short) is a low-carb, high-fat diet that gives many health benefits.

Over 25 studies show that this sort of diet could assist you to lose to weight and advance your health.

Ketogenic diets could even have advantages against diabetes, cancer, epilepsy, and Alzheimer's disease.

The ketogenic diet is a very low-carb, high-fat diet that has several comparisons with the Atkins and low-carb diets.

It comprises radically decreasing carbohydrate intake and supplanting it with fat. This decrease in carbs puts your body into a metabolic state termed ketosis.

When this occurs, your body becomes extremely effective at burning fat for energy. It also turns fat into ketones in the liver, which could provide good energy for the brain.

Ketogenic diets could cause enormous reductions in blood sugar and insulin levels. This, along with the enhanced ketones, has abundant health benefits.

NOTE: The keto diet is a low-carb, high-fat diet. It reduces blood sugar and insulin levels, and alter the body's metabolism away from carbs and towards fat and ketones.

## 1.1 Different Types of Ketogenic Diets

There are numerous varieties a of the ketogenic diet, comprising:

• A standard ketogenic diet (SKD): This is precisely a low-carb, moderate protein, and high-fat diet. It usually has 70% fat, 25% protein, and merely 5% carbs.

• A cyclical ketogenic diet (CKD): This diet comprises stages of higher-carb refeeds, like 5 ketogenic days followed by 2 high-carb days.

• A targeted ketogenic diet (TKD): This diet permits you to enhance carbs around workouts.

• High-protein ketogenic diet: This is related to a standard ketogenic diet. However, it contains more protein. The ratio is always 65% fat, 30% protein, and 5% carbs.

Conversely, simply the standard and high-protein ketogenic diets have been studied comprehensively. Cyclical or targeted ketogenic diets are more cutting-edge methods and principally used by bodybuilders or athletes.

We will talk mostly on the standard ketogenic diet (SKD), even though many of the same philosophies also apply to the other types.

NOTE: There are numerous versions of the keto diet. The standard (SKD) version is the most investigated and most recommended.

## 1.2 Ketogenic Diets Can Assist You Lose Weight

A ketogenic diet is an efficient approach to lose weight and lesser risk factors for disease.

Research indicates that the ketogenic diet is more superior to the frequently suggested low-fat diet.

What's more, the diet is so satisfying that you could lose weight without counting calories or tracking your food consumption.

One study found that individuals on a ketogenic diet lost 2.3 times more weight than those on a calorie-restricted low-fat diet. Triglyceride and HDL cholesterol levels also enhanced.

Another study found that folks on the ketogenic diet lost 3 times more weight than those on a diet suggested by Diabetes UK.

There are many reasons why a ketogenic diet is superior to a low-fat diet, comprising the increased protein intake, which offers many advantages.

The improved ketones, lower blood sugar levels and enhanced insulin sensitivity might also play a crucial role.

NOTE; A ketogenic diet could assist you to lose much more weight than a low-fat diet. This habitually ensues without hunger.

### 1.3Ketogenic Diets for Diabetes and Prediabetes

Diabetes is described by changes in metabolism, high blood sugar, and reduced insulin function.

The ketogenic diet can assist you to lose extra fat, which is usually linked to type 2 diabetes, prediabetes, and metabolic syndrome.

One study found that the ketogenic diet enriched insulin sensitivity by a massive 75% .

Another study in persons with type 2 diabetes found that 8 of the 22 partakers were able to stop using all diabetes drugs.

In yet another study, the ketogenic group lost 24.6 pounds (11.2 kg), related to 15.4 pounds (7.0 kg) in the higher-carb group. This is a substantial advantage when considering the link between weight and type 2 diabetes.

## CHAPTERTWO

## Ketogenic diet foods – what you have to eat

Are you not assured of what to eat on a keto diet?

At this point, you would find a good food list , revealing what you what to eat and avoid on keto. Let's start with a basic outline:

In a nutshell, eat real low-carb foods such as meat, fish, eggs, vegetables and natural fats similar to butter or olive oil. As a primary learner's rule, stick to foods with less than 5% carbs (numbers above).

### 2.1 Shun These Foods

These are what you should not eat on a keto diet – foods full of sugar and starch. As you could see, these foods are much higher in carbs.

Drinks

Drink water, coffee, tea, or the occasional glass of wine.

Warning: This ebook is for adults with health challenges, comprising obesity, that could profit from a keto diet. Though the menu has established benefits, it's still contentious.

There might be a need to adapt pre-existing prescriptions — deliberate any changes in medication and related lifestyle changes with your doctor.

Moreover, 96.2% of the ketogenic group were also able to stop or lessen diabetes medication, linked to 63% in the higher-carb group.

NOTE; The ketogenic diet could increase insulin sensitivity and cause fat loss, leading to substantial health benefits for folks with type 2 diabetes or prediabetes.

## 2.2 Full keto diet food list

- Meat – Untreated meats are low carb, and keto-friendly and organic and grass-fed meat might even be in good health.

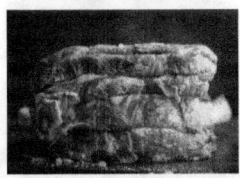

- But then, recall that keto is a high-fat diet, not high protein. Thus, you don't need vast amounts of meat. Extra protein (more than your body requires) is transformed into glucose, making it harder to get into ketosis.

-

- A reasonable amount of meat is sufficient.

Note: that processed meats, like sausages, cold cuts, and meatballs habitually contain added carbs. When in doubt look at the constituents, go for under 5% carbs.

- Fish and seafood – These are all good, particularly fatty fish like salmon. Conversely, avoid breading, as it comprises carbs. If you could find wild-caught fish that's perhaps the

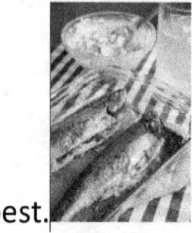

best.

- Eggs – Eat them any way, e.g., cooked, fried in butter, scrambled or as omelets, whatever

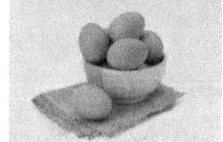

you need.

Purchasing organic or pastured eggs might be a better option.

How many eggs can you eat, bearing in mind cholesterol? Our recommendation is no more than 36 eggs each day.

Nevertheless, feel free to eat fewer if you wish.

- Natural fat, high-fat pastes – Most of the calories on a keto diet should come from fat. You'll be expected to get much of it from natural sources such as meat, fish, eggs, etc. Nevertheless, use fat in cooking, such as butter or coconut fat, and add sufficiently of olive oil to salads, etc.

You could also eat pleasant high-fat sauces containing Bearnaise sauce etc., or garlic butter (recipes).

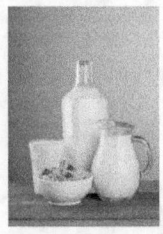

Recall, don't fear fat.

- Vegetables are growing above ground. Fresh or frozen – both are fine. Select plants growing above ground (here's why), particularly leafy and green items. Preferences include cauliflower, cabbage, avocado, broccoli, and zucchini.

Vegetables are an excellent and tasty means to eat good fat on keto. Fry them in butter and pour sufficient olive oil on your salad.

Some even consider vegetables as a fat-delivery system. They also add additional diversity, flavor, and color to your keto meals.

Several people end up eating more vegetables than before when starting keto, as veggies supplant the pasta, rice, potatoes, etc.

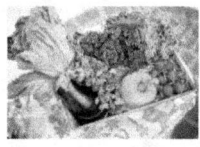

• High-fat dairy – Butter is good, high-fat cheese is okay, and high-fat yogurts can be had in moderation.

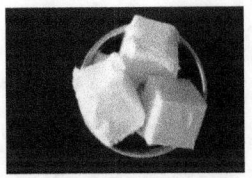

- Heavy cream is decent for cooking.

Avoid drinking milk as the milk sugar rapidly adds up (one glass = 15 grams of carbs). Moreover, you could use it cautiously in your coffee. Indeed shun caffè latte(18 grams of carbs). Also sidestep low-fat yogurts, mainly as they frequently contain lots of added sugars.

To conclude, be aware that habitually snacking on cheese when you're not hungry.

,

- Nuts – Can be had in moderation, though, be cautious when using nuts as snacks, as it's very cool to eat far more than you need to feel fulfilled. Also, be conscious that cashews are comparatively high carb, choose macadamia or pecan nuts.

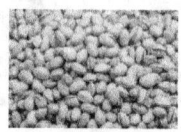

• Berries – A reasonable amount is OK on keto, possibly with real whipping cream, a typical keto dessert.

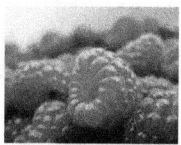

Drink

• Water – The #1 preference. Have it flat, with ice, or glittering. Drink it hot like a tea, or add natural flavorings such as sliced cucumbers, lemons, or limes. If you experience headaches or signs of "keto flu," add a few shakes of salt to your water.


• Coffee – No sugar. A small quantity of milk or cream is sufficient. For extra energy from fat, stir in butter and coconut oil for "Bulletproof coffee." Note, if weight loss reduces, cut back on the cream or fat in your coffee.

• Tea – Whether black, green, Orange Pekoe, mint, or herbal — make sure to drink most beverages. Don't add sugar.


• Bone broth – Hydrating, substantial, full of nutrients and electrolytes — and simple to make! — Homemade bone broth could be a unique beverage to sip on the keto diet. Stir in a pat of butter for some additional energy.

## CHAPTER THREEE

## High-carb foods to circumvent

- Sugar: This is what you mustn't even touch. Stop taking all soft drinks, fruit juice, sports drinks and "vitamin water" (these are all essentially sugar water).

Shun sweets, candy, cakes, cookies, chocolate bars, donuts, frozen treats, and breakfast cereals.

Always read labels for concealed sugars, particularly in sauces, condiments, drinks, dressings and packaged goods. Honey, maple syrup, and agave are also sugars. Preferably try to circumvent or limit non-natural sweeteners as well.

- Starch: Bread, pasta, rice, potatoes (as well as sweet potatoes), French fries, potato chips, porridge, muesli, and so on. Stop wholegrain products as well.

Legumes, like beans and lentils, are very high in carbs too. Small amounts of some root

Vegetables (other than potatoes and sweet potatoes) might be OK.

Note that there are several suitable replacements for these foods, that work on a keto diet. These are some of them:

– Keto bread

– Keto "pasta."

– Keto "rice."

– Keto porridge

• Beer: Liquid bread. Complete of quickly absorbed carbs. But there are a few lower-carb beers

• Fruit: Very sweet, lots of sugar. Eat it once in a while. Treat fruit as a natural form of candy.

### 3.1 Foods to Avoid

Any food that is high in carbs should be restricted.

These are a list of foods that need to be reduced or eradicated on a ketogenic diet:

- Sugary foods: fruit juice, chocolates, cake, ice cream, candy, etc.

- Grains or starches: Wheat-based foodstuffs, like rice, pasta, cereal, etc.

- Fruit: All fruit, except for small rations of berries like strawberries.

- Beans or legumes: Peas, kidney beans, lentils, chickpeas, etc.

- Root vegetables and tubers: Potatoes, sweet potatoes, carrots, spinach, etc.

- Low-fat or diet products: These are extremely processed and habitually high in carbs.

- Some condiments or sauces: These always have sugar and unhealthy fat.

- Unhealthy fats: Restrict your consumption of treated vegetable oils, mayonnaise, etc.

- Alcohol: Owing to their carb content, several alcoholic beverages could throw you out of ketosis.

- Sugar-free diet foods: These are usually high in sugar alcohols, which could affect ketone levels in many cases. These foods also used to be highly processed.

NOTE. Shun carb-based foods such as grains, sugars, legumes, rice, potatoes, candy, juice, and even several fruits.

### 3.2   Foods to Eat

You should base the bulk of your meals around these foods:

• Meat: Red meat, lean meat, ham, sausage, chicken, and turkey.

• Fatty fish: Like salmon, trout, tuna, and mackerel.

• Eggs: Go for pastured or omega-3 whole eggs.

• Butter and cream: Go for grass-fed when possible.

• Cheese: Unrefined cheese (cheddar, cream, blue or mozzarella).

• Nuts and seeds: Almonds, walnuts, flax seeds, pumpkin seeds, etc.

• Healthy oils: Largely extra virgin olive oil, coconut oil, and avocado oil.

- Avocados: Whole avocados or newly made

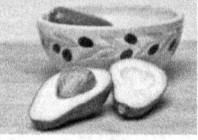

guacamole.

- Low-carb veggies: Many green vegetables, tomatoes, onions, peppers, etc.

- Condiments: You could use salt, pepper, and several healthy herbs and spices.

It is better to base your diet regularly on the whole, single-ingredient foods.

NOTE: Base the bulk of your diet on foods like meat, fish, eggs, butter, nuts, healthy oils, avocados and ample of low-carb veggies.

## CHAPTER FOUR

## Healthy Keto Snacks

Assuming, you get hungry between meals; these are some healthy, keto-approved snacks:

- Fatty meat or fish

- Cheese

- A bit of nuts or seeds

- Cheese with olives

- 1–3 hard-boiled eggs

- 92% dark chocolate

- A low-carb milkshake with the combination of almond milk, cocoa powder, and nut butter

- Whole-fat yogurt thoroughly mixed with nut butter and cocoa powder

- Strawberries and cream

- Celery with salsa and guacamole

- Less significant portions of leftover meals

NOTE; Great snacks for a keto diet comprises of pieces of meat, cheese, olives, boiled eggs, nuts, and dark chocolate.

## 4.1 A Sample Keto Meal Plan For 1 Week

To assist you in getting started, these are samples ketogenic diet meal plan for one week:

Monday

- Breakfast: Bacon, boiled eggs, and tomatoes.

- Lunch: Chicken salad thoroughly mixed with olive oil and feta cheese.

- Dinner: Salmon with asparagus prepared in butter.

Tuesday

- Breakfast: Egg, tomato, and goat cheese omelet.

- Lunch: Almond milk, peanut butter, cocoa powder, and a milkshake.

- Dinner: Meatballs, cheddar cheese, and vegetables.

Wednesday

- Breakfast: A ketogenic milkshake (attempt this or that).

- Lunch: Shrimp salad mixed with olive oil and avocado.

- Dinner: Pork chops with Parmesan cheese, broccoli, and lettuce.

Thursday

- Breakfast: Omelet with avocado, salsa peppers, onion, and different spices.

- Lunch: A bit of nut and celery sticks with guacamole and salsa.

- Dinner: Chicken sated with pesto and cream cheese, alongside vegetables.

Friday

- Breakfast: Sugar-free yogurt with peanut butter, cocoa powder, and stevia spices.

- Lunch: Beef stir-fry roasted in coconut oil with vegetables.

- Dinner: Bun-less burger with tasty bacon, egg, and cheese.

Saturday

- Breakfast: Ham and cheese omelet with vegetables.

- Lunch: Ham and cheese slices with different nuts.

- Dinner: Whitefish, egg, and spinach boiled in coconut oil.

Sunday

- Breakfast: Fried eggs with tasty bacon and mushrooms.

- Lunch: Burger with salsa, cheese, and guacamole.

- Dinner: Steak and eggs with a delicious salad.

At all times, try to alternate the vegetables and meat over the long term, as each kind offers different nutrients and health benefits.

## 4.2 Instructions for Eating Out on a Ketogenic Diet

It is not very hard to make many restaurant meals keto-friendly when eating out.

Several restaurants give some kind of meat or fish-based dish. Order this, and swap any high-carb food with additional vegetables.

Egg-based meals are also the right choice, like omelet or eggs and bacon.

A new favorite is bun-less burgers. You could also substitute the fries for vegetables in its place. Add extra avocado, cheese, bacon or eggs.

At Mexican restaurants, you could relish any type of meat with extra cheese, guacamole, salsa, and sour cream.

For dessert, go for a mixed cheese board or berries with cream.

NOTE; When eating out, pick a meat-, fish- or egg-based dish. Order additional veggies as a substitute of carbs or starches, and have cheese for dessert.

## CHAPTER FIVE

# Side Effects of Ketogenic Diet and How to Curtail Them

Though the ketogenic diet is safe for healthy people, there might be some initial side effects even though your body adjusts.

This is often referred to as the keto flu and is typically over inside a few days.

Keto flu comprises weak energy and mental function, increased hunger, sleep issues, nausea, digestive discomfort, and decreased exercise performance.

To reduce this, you could try a regular low-carb diet for the first few weeks. This might teach your body to burn more fat before you eradicate carbs.

A ketogenic diet could also alter the water and mineral balance of your body, so adding extra salt to your meals or taking mineral supplements could help.

For minerals, try taking 3,200–4,300 mg of sodium, 1,100 mg of potassium, and 350 mg of magnesium per day to reduce side effects.

At least, in the beginning, it is significant to eat up until you're full and avoid limiting calories too much. Generally, a ketogenic diet causes weight loss devoid of deliberate calorie restriction.

FOOTNOTE; Several of the side effects of starting a ketogenic diet can be inadequate. Easing into the food and taking mineral supplements could assist.

### 5.1    Supplements for a Ketogenic Diet

Even though no supplements are mandatory, some could be valuable.

•    MCT oil: Added to drinks or yogurt, MCT oil delivers energy and assists increase ketone levels.

•    Minerals: Extra salt and other minerals can be essential when beginning due to changes in water and mineral balance.

•    Caffeine: Caffeine could have benefits for energy, fat loss, and performance.

•    Exogenous ketones: This supplement might help raise the body's ketone levels.

•    Creatine: Creatine provides numerous benefits for health and performance. This can aid you if you are combining a ketogenic diet with exercise.

• Whey: Use half a scoop of whey protein in shakes or yogurt to increase your everyday protein intake.

NOTE; Some supplements could be useful on a ketogenic diet. These comprise of exogenous ketones, MCT oil, and minerals.

## 5.2 How low carb is keto?

Keto is a low-carb diet, not "no carb." So how much of carbs could you eat in a day?

The answer is that it depends. However, as a rough guide stay under 23 grams per day for maximum result, and if you love some benefit of low-carb eating (like weight loss),

you should possibly aim for at least staying under 122 grams of carbs per day.

Who should NOT do a ketogenic diet?

There are debates and myths about a keto diet, though for most individuals it seems to be very harmless.

There are, however, three groups that frequently need distinct attention:

- Do you take a drug for diabetes, e.g., insulin?
- Do you take a prescription for high blood pressure?
- Are you breastfeeding?

## •5.3    A Ketogenic Diet Is Exceptional, though Not for Everyone

A ketogenic diet is excellent for individuals who are overweight, diabetic, or looking to advance their metabolic health.

It might be less appropriate for elite athletes or those wanting to add large amounts of muscle or weight.

And, as with any diet, it would only work if you are consistent and stick with it for the long term.

That being said, few things are as well established in nutrition as the potent health and weight loss benefits of a ketogenic diet.

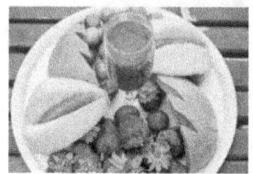

# CHAPTER SIX

# Uses and Benefits of the Ketogenic Diet

Whenever you are using a ketogenic diet, your body turns out to be more of a fat burner than a carbohydrate-dependent machine.

Several kinds of research have associated the ingestion of increased amounts of carbohydrates to the development of several disorders such as diabetes and insulin resistance.

By nature, carbohydrates are indeed absorbable and thus could also be effortlessly stored by the body. Digestion of carbohydrates starts right from the point you put them into your mouth.

As soon as you begin chewing them, scrutinize (the enzymes that digest carbohydrate) in your saliva is even now at work acting on the carbohydrate-containing food.

In the stomach, carbohydrates are further broken down. As soon as, they get into the small intestines, they are then absorbed into the bloodstream.

On getting to the bloodstream, carbohydrates habitually increase the blood sugar level.

This rise in blood sugar level encourages the prompt release of insulin into the bloodstream. The higher the increase in blood sugar levels, the more the amount of insulin that is released.

Insulin is a hormone that causes leftover sugar in the bloodstream to be removed to lower the blood sugar level.

Insulin takes the sugar and carbohydrate that you eat and stores them either as glycogen in muscle tissues or as fat in adipose tissue for future use as energy.

Furthermore, the body can advance what is known as insulin resistance when it is continually exposed to such high volumes of glucose in the bloodstream.

This condition can merely cause obesity as the body tends to store any excess amount of glucose quickly. Health conditions like diabetes and cardiovascular disease can also be the outcome of this circumstance.

Keto diets are low in carbohydrate and high in fat and have been linked with reducing and improving several health conditions.

One of the leading things a ketogenic diet does is to stabilize your insulin levels and also restore leptin signaling.

Reduced amounts of insulin in the bloodstream make you feel fuller for a lengthier period and also to have fewer cravings.

## 6.1 Medical Advantages of Ketogenic Diets

The application and implementation of the ketogenic diet have extended significantly. Keto diets are often stated as part of the treatment plan in several medical conditions.

### Epilepsy

This is basically the principal reason for the development of the ketogenic diet. For some reason, the degree of epileptic seizures reduces when patients are placed on a keto diet.

Pediatric epileptic cases are the most responsive to the keto diet. Some children have witness seizure elimination after a few years of using a keto diet.

Children with epilepsy are typically projected to fast for a few days before beginning the ketogenic diet as part of their treatment.

Cancer

Research supports that the therapeutic efficacy of the ketogenic diets against tumor growth can be enhanced when combined with some drugs and procedures under a "press-pulse" paradigm.

It is also conceivable to note that ketogenic diets drive the cancer cell into diminution. This implies that keto diets "starve cancer" to reduce the symptoms.

Alzheimer Disease

There are several signs that the memory functions of patients with Alzheimer's disease rise after making use of a ketogenic diet.

Ketones are a dependable source of alternative energy for the brain, mostly when it has become resilient to insulin.

Ketones also give substrates (cholesterol) that help to reestablish dented neurons and membranes. These also help to advance memory and cognition in Alzheimer patients.

## Diabetes

It is generally agreed that carbohydrates are the main culprit in diabetes. Therefore, by decreasing the amount of consumed carbohydrate using a ketogenic diet, there are better chances for enhanced blood sugar control.

Similarly, combining a keto diet with other diabetes treatment plans can considerably increase their overall effectiveness.

## Gluten Allergy

Numerous individuals with a gluten allergy are undiagnosed with this condition. Furthermore, following a ketogenic diet revealed progress in related symptoms such as digestive discomforts and bloating.

Most carbohydrate-rich foods are superb in gluten. Therefore, by using a keto diet, a lot of the gluten intake is reduced to a minimum owing to the elimination of a large selection of carbohydrates.

## Weight Loss

This is possibly the most common "intended" use of the ketogenic diet these days.

It has found a niche for itself in the current dieting trend. Keto diets have become part of many dieting regimens due to its well-recognized side effect of helping weight loss.

Even though initially smeared by many, the growing number of acceptable weight loss results has supported the ketogenic to better included as a leading weight loss program.

In addition to the aforementioned medical benefits, ketogenic diets also give some comprehensive health benefits which comprise the following.

Improved Insulin Sensitivity

This is obviously the first objective of a ketogenic diet. It assists in stabilizing your insulin levels, therefore, promoting fat burning.

Muscle Conservation

Ever since protein is oxidized, it helps to preserve lean muscle. Losing lean muscle mass makes an individual's metabolism to slow down as tissues are typically very metabolic. Using a keto diet truly aids to preserve your muscles while your body burns fat.

Precise pH and respiratory function

A keto diet assists to lessen lactate hence improving both pH and respiratory function. A state of ketosis, as a result, helps to hold your blood pH at a healthy level.

## Enhanced Immune System

Making use of a ketogenic diet helps to fight off aging antioxidants whereas also decreasing inflammation of the gut, thus making your immune system stronger.

## Reduced Cholesterol Levels

Eating fewer carbohydrates even though you are on the keto diet, will assist in diminishing blood cholesterol levels. This is due to the enriched state of lipolysis. This leads to a reduction in LDL cholesterol levels and a rise in HDL cholesterol levels.

## CHAPTER SEVEN

# The Advantages of Mixing MCT Oil into Your Ketogenic Diet Plan

In life, we're regularly talking about must-haves. If you're driving a high-end car, you have to have the top of the line motor oil flowing through its cylinders.

If you're challenging at a high level in a track competition, state of the art spike(running) shoes is a necessity. When you're rejoicing at a massive quarter at the office, the finest bourbon is a must have.

I would be obedient to you, that if you're serious about a ketogenic way of life, MCT Oil is a must-have.

MCT Oil gives a heavy dose of the very fuels that turn your body into - and retain it - a fat burning machine. Unlike LCTs, MCTs sidestep much of the digestion route that others fats go through.

MCTs act in an almost carb-like manner in how they're sent straight to the liver, where they are used for energy.

There are many reasons why MCT makes perfect sense for your Ketogenic Diet, but assist you in understanding how they could play a vital role in your nutrition; we've some of the significant benefits of MCT Oil in your Ketogenic Diet plan.

## 7.1 MCT OIL ASSIST YOUR GET INTO KETOSIS FASTER

As you already recognize, MCTs go to your liver and work in a "carb-like" manner that LCTs cannot do. This means that you can kick start Ketosis by following these steps:

1. Fast with no breakfast.

If you've been out of Ketosis for a while and you wish to get back into a fat burning state ably, a mix of fasting and MCT Oil will do the job.

Just eat a meager carb dinner, or even shun dinner, and then wake up and don't eat breakfast! In its place, drink a cup of coffee, and put a tablespoon or two of MCT Oil into your coffee and sip it.

The shot of MCT, plus the already fasted state of your body, will have you back into Ketosis faster than if you tried to just steadily eat your way back into Ketosis (i.e., dietary Ketosis).

It's also worth noting that the energy you get from the MCT Oil and the coffee will be different from what you were used to the MCTs offer sustained the energy that isn't equivalent to energy obtained from glycogen.

## 7.2. Meal replacement with MCT Oil

Another advantage that comes from using MCT Oil in your Ketogenic Diet plan is using it as a meal replacement.

This, to some extent, looks like the previous point of fasting with MCT Oil.

Nevertheless, the difference is that you're still eating other regular Ketogenic meals, except if you are switching (at least) one of those meals with roughly some MCT Oil.

One of the benefits of MCT Oil is its ability to satisfy your appetite. Thus while it sounds at first scary to just depend on a few tablespoons of oil for a meal replacement, your body will become used to it as you do it more and more.

The MCTs will act as a replacement for what's typically there (glycogen), and your fierce-badger-hunger yearnings will reduce.

In our fast-paced, 21st century way of life, the benefits of being able to stay in Ketosis while only swigging a few tablespoons of MCTs cannot be overstated.

### 7.3 Ramp up your Ketogenic dishes with MCT

MCT Oil's usefulness is fantastic. Let's say you're presently in Ketosis.

However, you're about to eat a salad for your daily carbs, and you like to keep it 100 on the Keto life.

It's cool! Just make use of MCT for a base to your dressing, and you could rest assured that you'll still be burning fat after you've put down your greens!

Another means to use MCTs in your favorite Ketogenic meals is to use it as a replacement for regular oil in baking!

There's an entire ocean of Keto baking recipes out there, so why not double down and use MCT as a substitute to regular coconut oil?!

But then, what if you're not baking? What if you're out for a jog and you wish to implement the energy productivity of MCT Oil? How about a sweet Keto "sports drink"?!

All you have to do is to water, and then have some lemon juice, and you'll have a better, non-sugary sports drink for long workouts in the sun!

There are numerous ways to skin a cat, and there are also several ways to reinforce your Ketogenic Diet.

MCTs are needed for your body transmuting into a fat burning machine. Unfortunately, you're not frequently going to be able to get the proper amounts from a diet alone - you'll need a boost, and MCT Oil is that lift.

Life is full of "must haves," and your diet does not fall out of the realm of this mantra.

If you wish to live a strictly Ketogenic lifestyle, you're going to have to spend on the right fuels and implement them in the most effective ways possible.

So what's the advantage of MCT to your Ketogenic Diet strategy? The answer: is efficiency.

An effective diet, which feeds a productive lifestyle, that eventually gives you more time to do the things you love.

Adopting a ketogenic diet helps you to decrease both your appetite and cravings for calorie-rich foods. As you commence eating healthy, sustaining, and valuable high-fat foods, your hunger feelings will certainly start reducing.

# CHAPTER EIGHT

## Other Health Benefits of Keto

The ketogenic diet actually started as a tool for treating neurological diseases such as epilepsy.

Studies have now shown that the diet can have benefits for a wide range of diverse health conditions:

• Heart disease: The ketogenic diet could enhance risk factors like body fat, HDL cholesterol levels, blood pressure, and blood sugar.

• Cancer: The diet is presently being used to treat numerous kinds of cancer and slow tumor growth.

• Alzheimer's disease: The keto diet might lessen symptoms of Alzheimer's disease and slow its progression.

• Epilepsy: Research has shown that the ketogenic diet could cause enormous reductions in seizures in epileptic children.

• Parkinson's disease: One study found that the diet helped advance symptoms of Parkinson's disease.

- Polycystic ovary syndrome: The ketogenic diet can help decrease insulin levels, which might play a substantial role in polycystic ovary syndrome.

- Brain injuries: Some studies found that the diet can lessen concussions and aid recovery after brain injury.

- Acne: Lesser insulin levels and eating less sugar or treated foods could help improve acne.

### 8.1. Why Must you eat a keto diet – the health benefits

The gains of a ketogenic diet are comparable to those of other low-carb diets. Nevertheless, it seems to be more potent than liberal low-carb diets.

Think of keto as a super-charged low-carb diet, take full advantage of the benefits. Furthermore, it can also be harder to do, and it could raise the risk of side effects a bit.

Lose weight

Turning your body into a fat-burning machine can be valuable for weight loss. Fat burning is substantially increased, whereas insulin – the fat-storing hormone – levels drop significantly.

This seems to make it far easier for body fat loss to occur, without hunger.

More than 40 high-quality scientific studies show that, compared to other diets, low-carb and keto diets result in more effective weight loss.

Appetite control

On a keto diet, you're expected to gain new control over your appetite. When your body burns fat 24-7, it has perpetual access to weeks or months of stored energy, considerably reducing feelings of hunger. It's a ubiquitous experience, and studies demonstrate it.

This makes it easy to eat less and lose excess weight – just wait till you're hungry before you eat.

It also makes intermittent fasting easier, something that can super-charge efforts to reverse type 2 diabetes and speed up weight loss, beyond the effect of keto only.

Plus, you'll save tons of time and money by not having to eat snack all the time. Numerous people only feel the necessity to eat twice a day on a keto diet (always skipping breakfast), and some just once a day.

Not having to fight feelings of hunger could also possibly help with problems like sugar or food addiction, and probably some eating disorders, like bulimia, as well.

At least feeling fulfilled can be part of the solution. Food could stop being an enemy and become your friend – or simply fuel, whatsoever you desire.

## 8.2 Control blood sugar and reverse type 2 diabetes

A ketogenic diet supports control blood sugar levels. It is exceptional for managing type 2 diabetes, sometimes even leading to a total reversal of the disease. This has been established in studies.

It makes perfect sense since keto lowers blood-sugar levels, decreases the need for medications, and reduces the potentially harmful effect of high insulin levels.

As a keto diet may even reverse popular type 2 diabetes, it's possible to be effective at preventing it or reversing pre-diabetes.

Enhanced health markers

Many studies are showing that low-carb diets advance several essential risk factors for heart disease, comprising the cholesterol profile (HDL, triglycerides), while total cholesterol and LDL levels are typically impacted relatively modestly.

It's also typical to see increased blood sugar levels, insulin levels, and blood pressure.

These usually improved markers are linked to something called "metabolic syndrome," and improvements in weight, waist circumference, diabetes type 2 reversal, etc.

## Energy and mental performance

Some individuals use ketogenic diets precisely for increased mental performance. Also, it's common for folks to experience an increase in energy when in ketosis.

On keto, the brain doesn't require dietary carbs. It's driven 24-7 by ketones, an efficient brain fuel.

Hence, ketosis results in a steady flow of fuel (ketones) to the brain, thus evading complications experienced with big blood sugar swings.

This might sometimes result in enhanced focus and concentration, and resolution of brain fog, with upgraded mental clarity.

On the other hand, keep in mind that study into many of these areas is far from being conclusive.

## CHAPTER NINE

## How to get into ketosis on a keto diet

These are the seven most essential things to raise your level of ketosis, ranked from most to least significant:

1.   Limit carbohydrates to 25 digestible grams per day or less – astringent low-carb or keto diet. Fiber does not have to be regulated; it might even be helpful for ketosis.

How much are 25 grams of carbs?  Or just use our keto recipes and meal plans, they are intended to keep you under 25 grams with no counting needed.

Note that quite often, just limiting carbs to deficient levels results in ketosis. So this may be all you have to do. But the rest of the list below will help make sure that you're successful.

2.   Regulate protein to moderate levels. On a ketogenic diet, you should eat the protein you

require, but not much more. This is because excess protein is transformed into glucose in the body, decreasing ketosis.

If possible, stay at about 1.6 gram of protein per day, per kg of body weight – nearly 110 grams of protein per day if you weigh 72 kilos (154 pounds).

A common mistake that stops folks from getting into ketosis is too much protein. Our keto recipes are intended with the right amount of protein.

3.   Eat enough fat to feel contented.

This is the massive difference between a keto diet and starvation, that also results in ketosis. A keto diet is viable, but fasting is not.

When starving, you're expected to feel tired and hungry and give up, but a ketogenic diet is sustainable and can make you feel great.

So eat enough to feel fulfilled, and if you're hungry all the time, you should perhaps add more fat to your meals (like more butter, more olive oil, etc.). These keto recipes have the needed fat incorporated.

4. Shun snacking when not hungry. Eating more frequently than you need, just eating for fun and because there's food around, decreases ketosis and slows down weight loss.

Though using keto snacks will decrease the damage, and is fine when you're hungry.

5. If needed, add intermittent fasting. For illustration, avoid breakfast and only eat during 8 hours of the day, fasting for 16 hours

(i.e., 16:8 fasting). This is very efficient at boosting ketone levels, as well as fast-tracking weight loss and type 2 diabetes reversal.

It's also typically easy to do on keto.

6.   Add exercise – adding any kind of physical activity even though you are on low carb can increase ketone levels reasonably.

It could also help speed up weight loss and diabetes type 2 reversal marginally.

Exercise is not required to get into ketosis, but it might be helpful.

7.   Sleep well enough – for most individuals at least seven hours per night on average – and keep stress under control.

Sleep deficiency and stress hormones elevate blood sugar levels, slowing ketosis, and weight loss a bit.

Plus, they might make it tougher to stick to a keto diet, and resist temptations.

Thus while handling sleep and stress will not get you into ketosis on its own, it's still good thinking about.

Note: To get into ketosis, limit carbs to deficient levels, preferably below 20 net carbs per day. That's a ketogenic diet, and it's by far the most significant thing for ketosis to occur.

Should you need to intensify the effect, implement more steps from the list above, starting from the top.

### 9.1 How to know you're in ketosis

After starting a ketogenic diet, how do you do if you're in ketosis? It's possible to measure it by testing urine, blood, or breath samples. Moreover, there are also revealing symptoms that entail no testing:

• Dry mouth and increased thirst. Except you drink enough and get enough electrolytes, like salt, you might feel a dry mouth. Try a cup of bouillon or two daily, plus as much water as you require. You may also sense a metallic taste in your mouth.

- Improved urination. A ketone body, acetoacetate, may end up in the urine. This makes it probable to test for ketosis using urine strips. It also – at least when starting – can result in having to go to the bathroom more regularly. This may be the chief cause of the increased thirst (above).

- Keto breathe. This is owing to a ketone body called acetone escaping through our breath.

 It could make a person's breath smell "fruity," or comparable to nail polish remover. This smell can occasionally also be felt from sweat when working out. It's habitually temporary.

Other, less specific but more positive signs comprise:

## •9.2 A Ketogenic Diet Is Exceptional, though Not for Everyone

A ketogenic diet is excellent for individuals who are overweight, diabetic, or looking to advance their metabolic health.

It might be less appropriate for elite athletes or those wanting to add large amounts of muscle or weight.

And, as with any diet, it would only work if you are consistent and stick with it for the long term.

That being said, few things are as well established in nutrition as the potent health and weight loss benefits of a ketogenic diet.

Whenever you are using a ketogenic diet, your body turns out to be more of a fat burner than a carbohydrate-dependent machine.

Several kinds of research have associated the ingestion of increased amounts of carbohydrates to the development of several disorders such as diabetes and insulin resistance.

By nature, carbohydrates are indeed absorbable and thus could also be effortlessly stored by the body. Digestion of carbohydrates starts right from the point you put them into your mouth.

As soon as you begin chewing them, scrutinize (the enzymes that digest carbohydrate) in your saliva is even now at work acting on the carbohydrate-containing food.

In the stomach, carbohydrates are further broken down. As soon as, they get into the small intestines, they are then absorbed into the bloodstream. On getting to the bloodstream, carbohydrates habitually increase the blood sugar level.

This rise in blood sugar level encourages the prompt release of insulin into the bloodstream. The higher the increase in blood sugar levels, the more the amount of insulin that is released.

Insulin is a hormone that causes leftover sugar in the bloodstream to be removed to lower the blood sugar level. Insulin takes the sugar and carbohydrate that you eat and stores them either as glycogen in muscle tissues or as fat in adipose tissue for future use as energy.

Furthermore, the body can advance what is known as insulin resistance when it is continually exposed to such high volumes of glucose in the bloodstream. This condition can merely cause obesity as the body tends to store any excess amount of glucose quickly. Health conditions like diabetes and cardiovascular disease can also be the outcome of this circumstance.

Keto diets are low in carbohydrate and high in fat and have been linked with reducing and improving several health conditions.

One of the leading things a ketogenic diet does is to stabilize your insulin levels and also restore leptin signaling. Reduced amounts of insulin in the bloodstream make you feel fuller for a lengthier period and also to have fewer cravings.

On the other hand, keep in mind that study into many of these areas is far from being conclusive.

Note: To get into ketosis, limit carbs to deficient levels, preferably below 20 net carbs per day. That's a ketogenic diet, and it's by far the most significant thing for ketosis to occur.

Should you need to intensify the effect, implement more steps from the list above, starting from the top.

## 9.3 Evaluating ketosis

There are three methods to measure ketones, which all come with pros and cons. Note that we have no relationships with any of the brands cited here.

1. Urine strips

2. Breath ketone analyzers

3. Blood ketone meter

### 1. Urine strips

Urine strips are the most straightforward and inexpensive way to measure ketosis. It is the first choice for most novices on a keto diet.

Dip the strip in your urine, and 15 seconds later, the color change will show you the presence of ketones.

If you get a high reading (a dark purple color), you'll recognize that you're in ketosis.

## 2. Breath-ketone analyzers

Breath-ketone analyzers are a modest way to measure ketones

In your breath, At $170 and up, they are more costly than urine strips. But they are low-priced than blood-ketone meters in the long run, as they are reusable any number of times.

These analyzers do not give you an exact ketone level when used on their own but offer a color code for the general level.

## 3. Blood-ketone meters

Blood-ketone meters show a particular and current level of ketones in your blood.

They are the gold standard and the most particular way to measure your ketosis level on a ketogenic diet. The major drawback, nevertheless, is that they are quite expensive, previously at least $2 per test.

Now it's probably to get cheaper tests.

## CHAPTER TEN

### How to get to optimal ketosis

Getting into ketosis on a ketogenic diet is not a black or white thing. It's not like you're either in ketosis or out of ketosis. In its place, you can be in different degrees of ketosis, as this chart demonstrates.

The numbers below denote the values when testing blood ketone levels.

- Below 0.5 mmol/l is not considered "ketosis," though a value of, say, 0.2 establishes that you're getting close. At this level, you're very much far away from extreme fat-burning.

- Between 0.5 – 1.5 mmol/l is light nourishing ketosis. You'll likely be getting a good effect on your weight, but maybe not optimal.

- Around 1.5 – 3 mmol/l is termed optimal ketosis and is sometimes suggested for maximum mental and physical performance gains.

It tends to make the most of fat burning, which might increase weight loss.

• Over 3 mmol/l is higher than necessary. It will possibly attain neither better nor worse results than being at the 1.5–3 level. Higher numbers can also sometimes mean that you're not getting sufficient food ("starvation ketosis"). For type 1 diabetics, it can be triggered by a severe lack of insulin that needs urgent attention.

• Over 8–10 mmol/l: It's usually impossible to get to this level just by eating a keto diet. It means that something is wrong. The most prevalent cause by far is type 1 diabetes, with severe deficiency of insulin.

Symptoms comprise feeling very sick with nausea, vomiting, abdominal pain, and confusion. The likely result, ketoacidosis, may be fatal and needs immediate medical care.

## 10.1 Keto flu

Most persons who start a ketogenic diet will witness some symptoms of the "keto flu." This is what you may sense, more or less, a few days after you've started a keto diet:

- Headache

- Exhaustion

- Dizziness

- Light nausea

- Difficulty focusing ("brain fog")

- Lack of motivation

- Irritability

These initial symptoms typically disappear in a week, as your body adjusts to increased fat burning.

The foremost cause of the keto flu is that carb-rich foods can result in water retention (swelling) in the body.

When you start a low-carb diet, much of this additional fluid is lost. You may notice increased urination, and with that, some added salt is lost too.

This can result in dehydration and a lack of salt before your body acclimatizes. This seems to be the reason behind most of the symptoms of the keto flu.

You can decrease or even eradicate these symptoms by making sure you get sufficient water and salt. One simple way to do this is to drink a cup of bouillon or broth, 1-2 times per

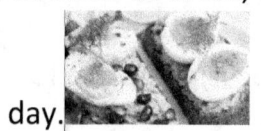

day.

## CHAPTER ELEVEN

## The keto diet recipe:

The keto diet is one of the most efficient that I've come across and one of the more straightforward (as opposed to easy!) to follow.

Moreover, when you're on a keto diet, you eat a very low-carb, high-fat diet. That means goodbye to pasta and bread, hello cheese and oils. It's much the opposite of what we've been taught our entire lives.

Though, it works if you follow the Plus, you can make numerous favorite recipes keto-friendly.

What makes the keto diet work correctly is that, with little glucose from carbohydrates in our bodies, we have to burn something else — fat — for energy. The keto diet can cause the body to burn fat quite speedily (hurray!).

Whether you're brand new to the keto diet or a seasoned vet, these keto recipes will fulfill your low carb diet needs. There are numerous variations of the keto diet, so be sure to double check the constituents before you cook.

1

Cheesy Cauliflower Breadsticks

These grain-free "breadsticks" are made with cauliflower as a substitute for flour. It's one of our preferred keto recipes! Serve with your favorite marinara sauce.—

2

Chicken & Goat Cheese Skillet

My husband was entirely bowled over by this on-a-whim skillet meal. I can't wait to make it again very soon! —

3

Carrot and Kale Vegetable Saute

Appreciations to garden-fresh veggie dishes like this one, I nearly overlook I'm wheat- and gluten-free. Bacon adds another layer of flavor and penetration to this stunning side dish. — Darla Andrews, Schertz, Texas.

4

Herbed Balsamic Chicken

Our kitchen is tiny and cramped, so we try to grill simple (but tasty) meals outside as always as possible during the summer months. Dried herbs work as well; however, during the summer use fresh herbs for the best taste. —

5

Garlic-Dill Deviled Eggs

In my immediate family, Easter isn't wholly devoid of deviled eggs. Fresh dill and garlic perk up the flavor of these mouthwatering appetizers you'll need to eat on every time. —

6

## Zucchini Crusted Pizza

Tasty, nutritious, and useful, this pizza is easy to prepare ahead and freeze—and fun to make with kids. It also quadruples pleasantly. What's not to like? —

## 7 /

## Creamy Dijon Chicken

This chicken dish is enormously fast and cost-effective. It produces a mild sauce that works well over brown rice or wide noodles. If you love extra sauce for leftovers, double the recipe. —

## 8

## Naked Fish Tacos

This is one of my husband's all-time beloved meals. I've even persuaded some friends to fish after eating this. I serve it with freshly prepared melon when it's in the season to stabilize the subtle heat of the cabbage mixture. —

9

## Denver Omelet Salad

I love this recipe—it's not your usual breakfast, though, it has all the right elements: easy, healthy, and fast. Turn your favorite omelet ingredients into a morning salad! —

10 /

## Balsamic Zucchini Saute

This super-fast sautéed zucchini recipe is tasty and only uses a few constituents, so it's refreshing to whip up as your entree is cooking. —

11

## Blackened Tilapia with Zucchini Noodles

I love speedy and bright meals like this one-skillet wonder. The way it tastes, you'd feel it takes a lot more effort, even though it goes from prep to dinner table in half an hour. The recipe works perfectly with any light fish or even shrimp. —

12

Deviled Egg Spread

I made use of this egg salad at a luncheon and had to have it. I pierced it up with pickled banana peppers. It's a hit with my children and picky mother. — .

13


Asparagus-Mushroom Frittata

My Sicilian, Aunt Paulina, encouraged this fluffy frittata. I recollect going to see her garden, harvesting fresh veggies and watching her cook. Her wild asparagus frittata was my beloved one. —

14

Blue Cheese Pork Medallions

This reassuring pork dish feels fancy, thanks to the creamy sauce kicked up a notch by blue cheese. Guests go crazy over it, and would never guess how speedily it all comes together. —

15

Asparagus & Cheese Frittata

This gorgeous and creamy frittata commences in the skillet and ends in the oven. We like this melty, cheesy dish with salad on the side. —

16

Oktoberfest Brats with Mustard Sauce

I come from a town with a great German heritage, and each year we have a massive celebration for Oktoberfest. This recipe packs in all the customary German flavors my whole family loves. —

17

Shrimp Avocado Salad

This salad can be served as a refreshing and sustaining dinner or lunch. The delicious taste and smooth texture of avocados mixed with the crisp shrimp salad are lovely. —

18

### Sage-Rubbed Salmon

If you've all the time thought of sage with turkey, try it with salmon for a little taste of heaven. We serve this with rice, salad, and sautéed green beans. —

19

### Cilantro Lime Shrimp

A rapid garlicky lime marinade works magic on these juicy shrimp. They come off the grill with massive flavors impeccable for your next cookout. —

20

### Parmesan Roasted Broccoli

Sure, it's healthy and straightforward; nevertheless, oh, is this roasted broccoli excellent. Cutting the stems into tall "trees" turns a regular veggie into a standout side dish. —

21

Smoky Cauliflower Bites

These healthy miniature treats work well as a side or as an entertaining appetizer. Roasting the cauliflower adds deep flavor and gives it an enticing crunch. —.

22


Avocado Crab Boats

These boats are delightful with tortilla chips, beans or rice. You could also cover them, pack them on ice, and take them to a picnic or potluck. Straight from the oven or cold, they're always pleasant. —.

23

Parmesan Chicken

The spicy coating on this chicken has the nourishing flavor of Parmesan cheese. It's easy enough to be a family weekday meal yet inspiring enough to serve to guests. Once I make this chicken for banquet, we never have remnants.

24

Roasted Parmesan Carrots

Mom persistently said, "eat your carrots, assist your eyes." Very Rich in beta carotene, carrots not only support health but also taste fantastic when roasted and tossed with Parmesan. —

25

Tangy Parmesan Tilapia

If you want a gluten-free fish coating, this works attractively! Some reduced-fat mayos may comprise gluten, though, so check the label on yours to be sure. —.

I have chosen how to prepare about 5 out of the 25 that I have highlighted above.

Chicken & Goat Cheese Skillet

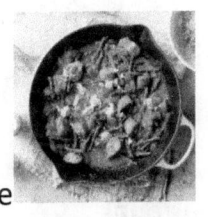

Total Time

Prep/Total Time: 22 min.

Makes

2 servings

Ingredients

- 1/3-pound boneless skinless chicken breasts, cut into 2-inch pieces

- 1/3 teaspoon salt

- 1/8 teaspoon pepper

- 3 teaspoons olive oil

- 1 cup chopped fresh asparagus (1-inch pieces)

- 1 garlic clove, minced

- 4 plum tomatoes, sliced

- 2 tablespoons 2% milk

- 3 tablespoons herbed fresh goat cheese, crushed

- Hot cooked rice or pasta

- Extra goat cheese, optional

Directions

- Toss chicken with salt and pepper. In a large skillet, heat oil over medium-high heat; saute chicken until no longer pink, 5-7 minutes. Take away from pan; keep warm.

- Add asparagus to skillet; cook and mix over medium-high heat 1 minute. Add garlic; cook and stir 32 seconds. Mix in tomatoes, milk and 2 tablespoons cheese; cook, covered, over medium heat till cheese starts to melt, 2-3 minutes. Stir in chicken. Serve with rice. If wanted, top with additional cheese.

Nutrition Facts

1-1/2 cups chicken mixture: 253 calories, 11g fat (4g saturated fat), 75mg cholesterol, 448mg sodium, 8g carbohydrate (5g sugars, 3g fiber), 29g protein. Diabetic Exchanges: 45lean meat, 3 fat, 1 vegetable.

Cheesy Cauliflower Breadsticks

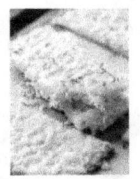

Total Time

Prep: 22 min. Bake: 32 min

Makes

12 servings

Ingredients

- 1 medium head cauliflower, cut into 1-inch florets (about 7 cups)

- 1/3 cup shredded part-skim mozzarella cheese

- 1/3 cup grated Parmesan cheese

- 1/3 cup shredded cheddar cheese

- 2 large egg

- 1/5 cup sliced fresh basil

- 1/5 cup cut fresh parsley

- 1 garlic clove, crushed

- 1 teaspoon salt

- 1/2 teaspoon pepper

- Marinara sauce, optional

## Directions

- Preheat oven to 426°. Process cauliflower in batches in a food processor till finely ground. Microwave, enclosed, in a microwave-safe bowl on high till tender, about 9 minutes.

When cauliflower is cool sufficiently to handle, wrap in a clean kitchen towel and squeeze dry. Return to bowl.

- In the meantime, in another bowl, mix cheeses. Blend half of the cheese mixture into cauliflower, reserving remainder. Combine next six ingredients; mix into the cauliflower.

- On a baking sheet lined with parchment paper, shape cauliflower mixture into an 11x9-in. Rectangle. Bake till edges are golden brown, 20-27 minutes. Top with reserved cheese; bake until melted and bubbly, 10-13 minutes.

Cut into 12 breadsticks. If wanted, serve with marinara sauce.

## Test Kitchen tips

• As long as you line your pan with parchment paper, these breadsticks can be made in any shape you love. A round pizza pan works kindly as well.

• Customize to your heart's wish by adding toppings such as pepperoni, mushrooms, and olives before baking.

## Nutrition Facts

1 breadstick: 67 calories, 5g fat (2g saturated fat), 27mg cholesterol, 342mg sodium, 5g carbohydrate (1g sugars, 1g fiber), 6g protein. Diabetic Exchanges: 1 medium-fat meat, 1 vegetable.


## Carrot and Kale Vegetable Saute

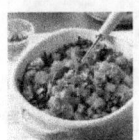

## Total Time

Prep: 18 min. Cook: 23 min

Makes

9 servings

Ingredients

- 9 bacon strips, coarsely chopped
- 5 large carrots, sliced
- 3cups peeled cubed butternut squash (1/2-inch pieces)
- 2 poblano pepper, seeded and chopped
- 1/2 cup excellently chopped red onion
- 2 teaspoon smoked paprika
- 1/5 teaspoon salt
- 1/5 teaspoon pepper
- 4 plum tomatoes, sliced
- 2 cups chopped fresh kale

Directions

- In a big skillet, cook bacon over medium heat until crispy, stirring intermittently. Using a slotted spoon, eliminate bacon to paper towels. Pour off all but 2 tablespoon drippings.

- Add carrots and squash to drippings; cook, covered over medium heat 6 minutes. Add poblano pepper and onion; cook until vegetables are soft, about 6 minutes, stirring sometimes. Stir in seasonings. Put tomatoes and kale; cook, well enclosed, till kale is wilting, 3-4 minutes. Top with bacon.

Test Kitchen Tips

- Use kitchen clippers to cut bacon into small pieces straight over the skillet.

- The sweet, rich flavor of smoked paprika is made by gradually drying peppers over a fire for some weeks.

- Poblano peppers are dark green and mild in flavor. When dried, they turn reddish black and are recognized as anchos.

Nutrition Facts

3/4 cup: 102 calories, 6g fat (3g saturated fat), 11mg cholesterol, 252mg sodium, 13g carbohydrate (5g sugars, 3g fiber), 4g protein.

Diabetic Exchanges: 2 vegetable, 2 fat, 1/2 starch.

## Herbed Balsamic Chicken

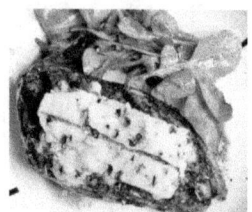

Total Time

Prep/Total Time: 33 min

Makes

8 servings

Ingredients

- 1/3 cup balsamic vinegar
- 4 tablespoons extra virgin olive oil
- 2 tablespoon minced fresh basil
- 2 tablespoon minced fresh chives
- 3 teaspoons grated lemon zest
- 2 garlic clove, minced

- 3/5 teaspoon salt

- 1/5 teaspoon pepper

- 7 boneless skinless chicken thighs (1-1/2 pounds)

Directions

- Whisk together all ingredients excluding chicken. In a bowl, toss chicken with 1/3 cup vinegar mixture; let stand 12 minutes.

- Grill chicken, enclosed, over medium heat or broil 4 in. From heat until a thermometer reads 172°, 7-9 minutes per side. Sprinkle with lingering vinegar mixture before serving.

Nutrition Facts

1 chicken thigh with 3 teaspoons sauce: 246 calories, 16g fat (4g saturated fat), 77mg cholesterol, 359mg sodium, 7g carbohydrate (5g sugars, 0 fiber), 21g protein. Diabetic Exchanges: 4 lean meat, 1-1/2 fat.

Garlic-Dill Deviled Eggs

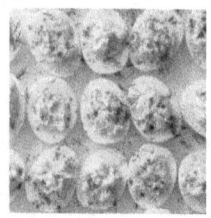

Total Time

Prep: 23 min. + chilling

Ingredients

- 13 large hard-boiled eggs

- 2/4 cup mayonnaise

- 5 teaspoons dill pickle relish

- 3 teaspoons cut fresh dill

- 3 teaspoons Dijon mustard

- 2 teaspoons coarsely ground pepper

- 1/5 teaspoon garlic powder

- 1/7 teaspoon paprika or cayenne pepper

Directions

- Cut eggs lengthwise in half. Get rid of yolks, preserving whites. In a bowl, mash yolks. Mix in all remaining ingredients apart from paprika. Spoon or pipe into egg whites.

- Refrigerate, covered, at least 32 minutes before serving. Sprinkle with paprika.

Nutrition Facts

1 stuffed egg half: 82 calories, 8g fat (2g saturated fat), 96mg cholesterol, 82mg sodium, 1g carbohydrate (0 sugars, 0 fiber), 4g protein.

Zucchini Crusted Pizza

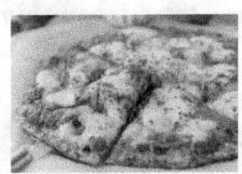

Total Time

Prep: 22 min. Bake: 26 min

Makes

8 servings

Ingredients

- 4 large eggs, lightly beaten

- 3cups shredded zucchini (about 1-1/2 medium), squeezed dry

- 1/3 cup shredded part-skim mozzarella cheese

- 1/3 cup grated Parmesan cheese

- 1/4 cup all-purpose flour

- 2 tablespoon olive oil

- 2 tablespoon crushed fresh basil

- 1 teaspoon crushed fresh thyme

- TOPPINGS:

- 1 jar (12 ounces) cooked sweet red peppers, julienned

- 1 cup shredded part-skim mozzarella cheese

- 1/3 cup cut turkey pepperoni

Directions

- Preheat oven to 452°. Mix first 9 ingredients; transfer to a 12-in. Pizza pan coated kindly with cooking spray. Spread mixture to an 11-in. Circle.

- Bake till light golden brown, 13-16 minutes. Lessen oven setting to 400°. Add toppings. Bake until cheese is molten, 10-13 minutes longer.

Nutrition Facts

1 slice: 220 calories, 14g fat (5g saturated fat), 97mg cholesterol, 682mg sodium, 12g carbohydrate (6g sugars, 1g fiber), 16g protein. Diabetic Exchanges: 3 medium-fat meat, 1 starch, 1 fat.

## Conclusion;

Life is full of "must haves," and your diet does not fall out of the realm of this mantra. If you wish to live a Ketogenic lifestyle, you're going to have to invest in the right fuels and implement them in the most effective ways possible.

So what's the advantage of MCT to your Ketogenic Diet plan? The answer: efficiency. An adequate diet, which feeds an active lifestyle, that eventually gives you more time to do the things you love.

The ketogenic diet can also be very pleasurable, with lovely fish, steaks, bacon, eggs, and fruit with cream on the menu. Enjoyment of food is vital if the diet is to prove justifiable.

Typically, low levels of complex carbohydrates will be re-introduced when excess weight has been shed for long term weight maintenance.